SOUL OF ZION
BODY OF OLYMPUS

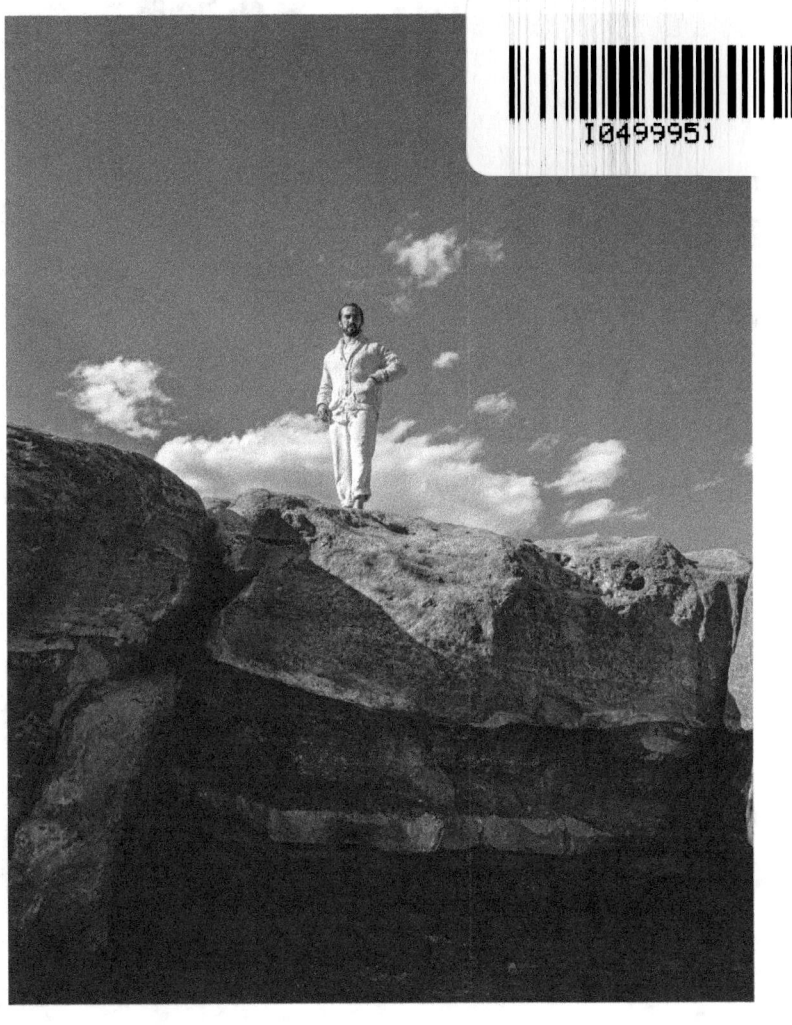

JOHN GOODHELM

LUX.GURU

SOUL OF ZION BODY OF OLYMPUS

BY JOHN GOODHELM

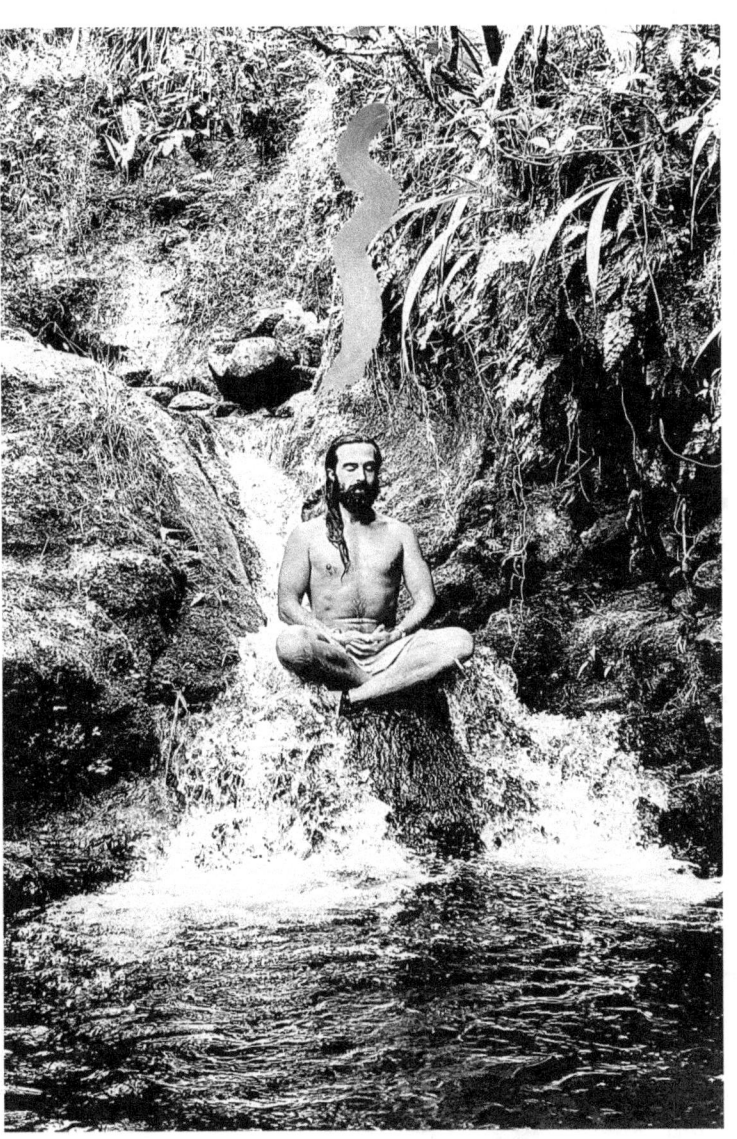

SOUL OF ZION

BODY OF OLYMPUS

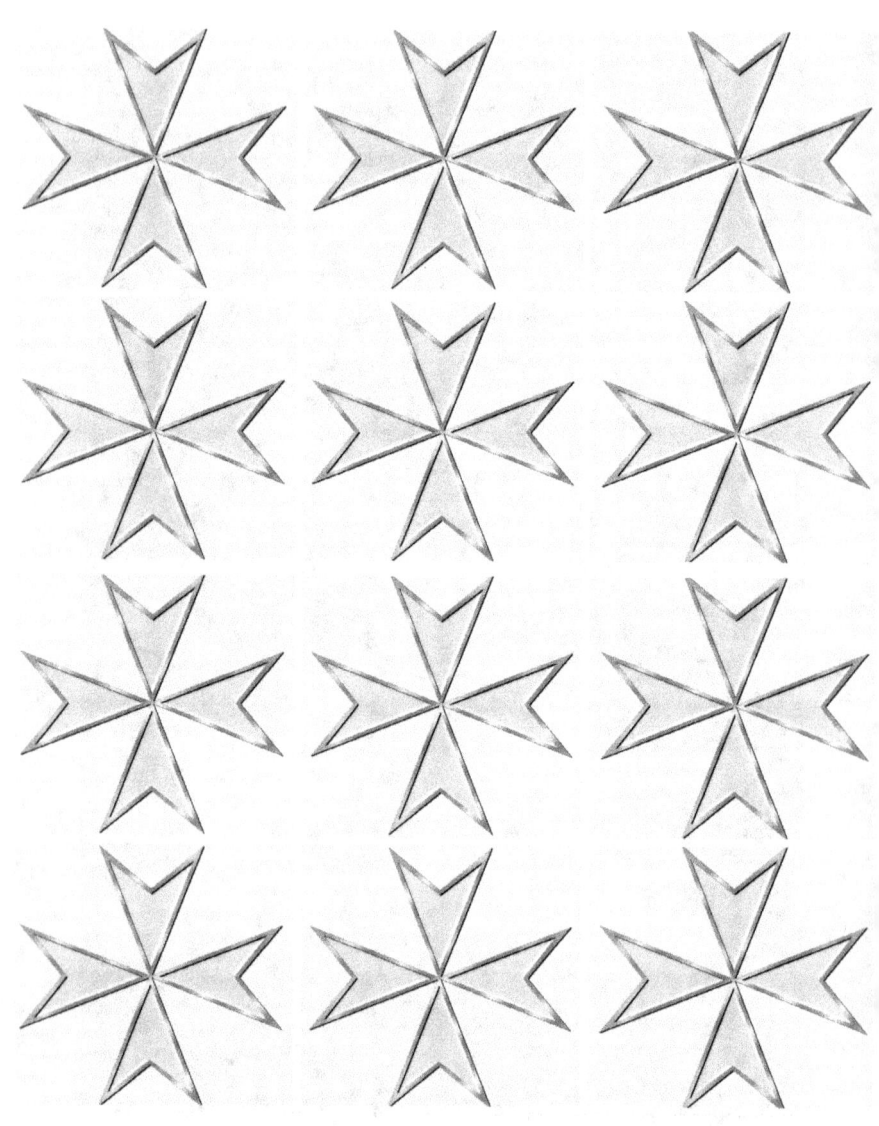

LUX.guru | Son of Light Ministry

A Global Ministry for the Revelation of Truth
'Glorify God Honor Self'

www.LUX.guru

To all who align their will with the thought of God; may we be as free in the body as out of it.

When the thunderous quakes come, and when the golden elixir flows, a sovereignty over self shepherds, all with thine mirable dictum, "Not my will, but thine; be done in me and through me," and the Light again has pierced the veil.

PROLOGUE

An overview of the concept of the Son of God from Adam to Jesus; this meta-physical blueprint and psychical guidebook shows how the spirit manifests vis-a-vis a description of all the parts unto the whole, that wholeness is the primary reality, and to be of one mind, one purpose in God.

The principles which paramount and inspire this books creation are oneness and unconditional love. Such ideals when looked to with a fixity of purpose give rise to a constellation of thoughts and their corresponding actions, and these too are the means by which this devotional is to take effect and reflect upon the reader an inclination towards the Divine. Diligo ergo sum.

For by so doing, an entrance shall be given freely to you into the everlasting kingdom of our LORD and Saviour Jesus Christ. Wherefore I will not be negligent to put you always in remembrance of these things, though you know them well; and you rely on this very truth. Therefore I think it is right, as long as I am in this body, to stir you up by putting you in remembrance; Knowing that shortly I must depart this life, even as our LORD Jesus Christ has shown me. Be diligent always, that you may be able to keep these things in remembrance; even after my departure.

-2nd Peter 1:11-15

ΓΝῶΘΙ ΣΕΑΥΤΟΝ (KNOW THYSELF)

Every new day is a new Genesis. There are 7 glands comprising the endocrine system which are analogous to and the mythic provenance of the seven days of creation recorded in the book of Genesis. The book of Revelation details the internal spiritual process of personal revelation and returning to creatorship - knowing and transcending self and in divine union.

יהי אור (LET THERE BE LIGHT)

GOD created the heavens and the earth in the very beginning. And the earth was without form, and void; and darkness was upon the face of the deep. And the Spirit of God moved upon the face of the water. And God said, Let there be light; and there was light.
   -Genesis 1:1-3

ΛΟΓΟΣ (TRUTH)

THE Word was in the beginning, and that very Word was with God, and God was that Word. The same was in the beginning with God. Everything came to be by his hand; and without him not even one thing came to be of what was created. The life was in him, and the life is the light of men. And the same light shines in the darkness, and the darkness does not overcome it.

-John 1:1-5

T hese are the experiences of souls as they entered
earth, an image in spirit to quicken freedom and
something to experience every day.

THE MIND OF GOD MOVED AND MATTER CAME INTO BEING

THE FIRST DAY
1. א.

And the earth was without form, and void; and darkness was upon the face of the deep. And the Spirit of God moved upon the face of the water. And God said, Let there be light; and there was light. And God saw that the light was good; and God separated the light from the darkness. And God called the light Day, and the darkness he called Night. And there was evening and there was morning, the first day.

-Genesis 1:2-5

EVERYDAY IS A NEW BEGINNING, A DAILY GENESIS AND BEGINNING FOR EVOLUTION.

THE SECOND DAY
2. ב.

And God said, Let there be a firmament in the midst of the waters, and let it divide the waters from the waters. And God made the firmament, and divided the waters that were under the firmament from the waters that were above the firmament; and it was so. And God called the firmament Sky. And there was evening and there was morning, the second day.
   -Genesis 1:6-8

SHIFTING CONSCIOUS AWARENESS AND AWAKENING

THE THIRD DAY
3. ג.

And God said, Let the waters that are under the sky be gathered together in one place, and let the dry land appear; and it was so. And God called the dry land Earth; and the gathering together of the waters he called Seas; and God saw that it was good. And God said, Let the earth bring forth vegetation, the herb yielding seed after its kind, and the fruit tree yielding fruit after its kind, wherein is their seed, upon the earth; and it was so. And the earth brought forth vegetation, the herb yielding seed after its kind, and the tree hearing fruit, wherein is its seed, after its kind; and God saw that it was good. And there was evening and there was morning, the third day.

-Genesis 1:9-13

THE DIMENSIONS OF CONSCIOUSNESS ON EARTH ARE WITH SEED WHICH PRODUCE THEIR OWN KIND

THE FOURTH DAY
4. ㅜ.

Then God said, Let there be lights in the firmament of the heaven to separate the day from the night; and let them be for signs, and for seasons, and for days, and years. And let them be for lights in the firmament of the heaven to give light upon the earth; and it was so. And God made two great lights, the greater light to rule the day, and the smaller light to rule the night; and the stars also. And God set them in the firmament of the heavens to give light upon the earth, And to rule over the day and over the night, and to separate the light from the darkness; and God saw that it was good. And there was evening and there was morning, the fourth day.
    -Genesis 1:14-19

THE SUN, MOON, AND STARS ARE SIGNS

THE FIFTH DAY
5. ה.

And God said, Let the waters bring forth swarms of living creatures, and let fowl fly above the earth in the open firmament of the heaven. And God created great sea monsters, and every living creature that moves, which the waters brought forth abundantly after their kind, and every winged fowl after its kind; and God saw that it was good. And God blessed them, saying, Be fruitful and multiply, and fill the waters in the seas, and let fowl multiply on the earth. And there was evening and there was morning, the fifth day.

-Genesis 1:20-23

SAVE LOST SOULS FROM ENMESHMENT IN MATERIALITY

THE SIXTH DAY
6. 1.

Then God said, Let the earth bring forth living creatures after their kind, cattle, and creeping things, and beasts of the earth after their kind; and it was so. And God made the beasts of the earth after their kind, and the cattle after their kind, and everything that creeps upon the earth after its kind; and God saw that it was good. Then God said, Let us make man in our image, after our likeness; and let them have dominion over the fish of the sea, and over the fowl of the air, and over the cattle, and over all the wild beasts of the earth, and over every creeping thing that creeps upon the earth. So God created man in his own image, in the image of God he created him; male and female he created them. And God blessed them, and God said to them, Be fruitful, and multiply, and fill the earth, and subdue it; and have dominion over the fish of the sea, and over the fowl of the air, and over the cattle, and over all the wild beasts that move upon the earth. And God said, Behold, I have given you every herb yielding seed, which is upon the face of all the earth, and every tree which bears fruit yielding seed; to you it shall be for food. And to every beast of the earth, and to every fowl of the air, and to everything that creeps upon the earth, wherein there is life, I have given every green herb for food; and it was so. And God saw everything that he had made, and, behold, it was very good. And there was evening and there was morning, the sixth day.

MALE AND FEMALE ARE AS ONE IN THE SPIRIT AND SEPARATE IN FLESH, AND AS SUCH BE FRUITFUL AND MULTIPLY.

Aware of duality in matter and the necessity for separate yet cooperative polarities, the Son of God in Adam is described. Later, Adam becomes the more perfect and immaculate concept of the Son of God, and as Jesus Christ is described.

THE SEVENTH DAY
7. ᴛ.

THUS the heavens and the earth were finished, and all the host of them. And on the sixth day God, finished his works which he had made; and he rested on the seventh day from all his works which he had made. So God blessed the seventh day, and sanctified it; because in it he had rested from all his works which God created and made.
   -Genesis 2:1-3

TAKE STOCK AND REST THAT HIS PURPOSE FLOWS THROUGH THAT MADE AND PERFECTED IN SELF

But, my beloved, do not forget this one thing, that one day is with the LORD as a thousand years, and a thousand years as one day.
-2 Peter 3:8

THE EARTH AND THE UNIVERSE CAME INTO BEING THROUGH THE MIND OF THE CREATOR

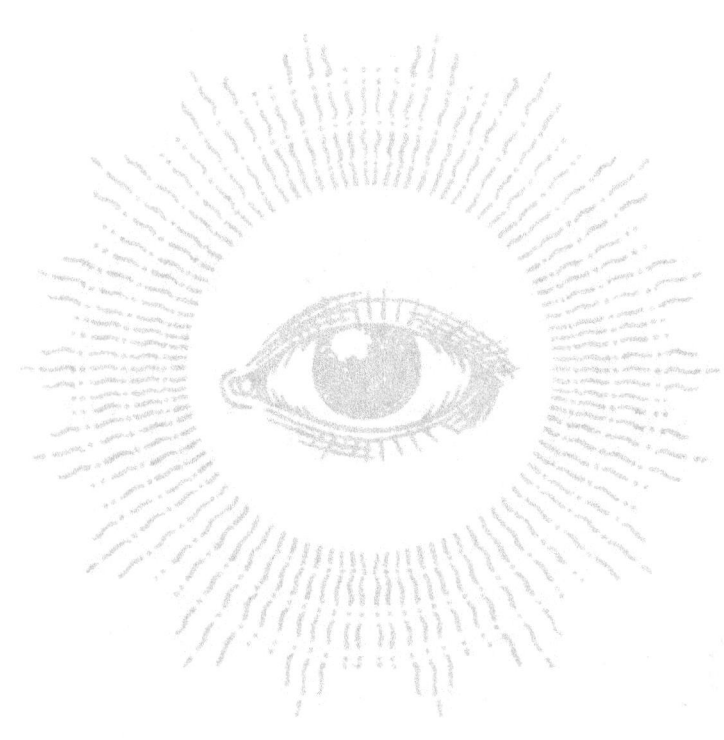

INTEGRATE, ALIGN, BE WHOLLY THE LIGHT; REBORN IN THE SPIRIT AND ONE WITH GOD

Revelation isn't the end, but the beginning. It is the story of a personal revelation and details the internal spiritual process to align with Christ as a Son of Light. Listed are 7 churches which correspond to the 7 glands of the endocrine system. These glands have a structural and functional correlation and are anatomically located in ascending revelatory order patterned in the shape of a shepherds crook. In this way Revelation is a pattern for self-awareness with holistic insight into the subtle physiology - physically indicated as 7 glands and as an integrated current, as a 'New Jerusalem' aligned with the love of God.

THE INNER FORCES WITHIN THE BODY ARE SPIRIT IN ACTION. WHEN WE SEEK TO BE ONE WITH HIM IN BODY, MIND, AND SOUL WE DRAW SPIRIT IN THE BODY AND COAGULATE ENERGY INTO A HIGHER PHYSICAL EXPRESSION.

John to the seven churches which are in Asia: Grace be to you, and peace, from him who is, and who was, and who is to come; and from the seven spirits which are before his throne.
-Revelation 1:4

Redirect the senses inward so that layers of transformation with internal balance and integration raise energy up the spine, passing through seven seals (glands), where one sits in Heaven next to 24 elders (cranial nerves). Self-aware do they read from the book of remembrance, a story of a celestial sojourn, and restored to the dignity of their creation do they read from the book of Life, as a Son of God.

These things says the Omnipotent; who holds the seven stars in his right hand, who walks in the midst of the seven golden candlesticks.
-Revelation 2:1

Set the ideal in the Christ, as lived by Jesus, a teacher who was bold; keep the light as your goal. An ideal requires aspiration and trust. All that strive gain. According to your faith be it unto you.

I am Alpha and Omega, the beginning and the ending says the LORD God, who is, and who was, and who is to come, the Almighty. I, John, your brother, and companion in suffering, and in the hope of Jesus Christ, was in the island which is called Patmos, because of the word of God, and because of the testimony of Jesus Christ. The Spirit of prophecy came upon me on the LORD'S day, and I heard behind me a great voice, as of a trumpet, saying, I am Alpha and Omega, the first and the last.
-Revelation 1:8-10

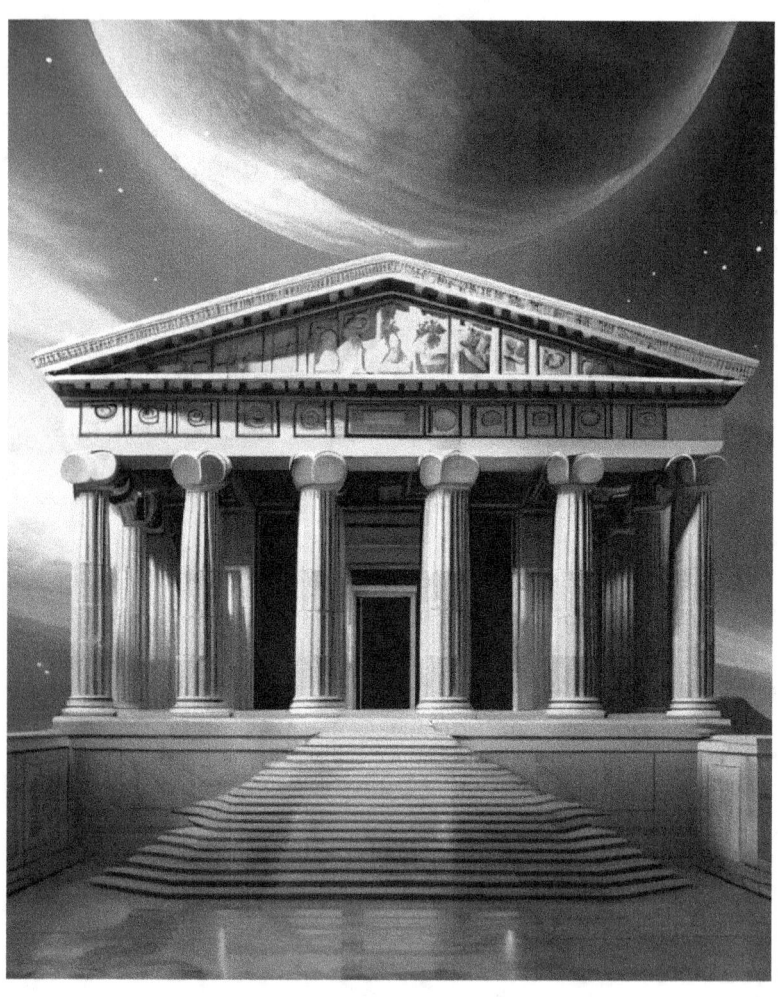

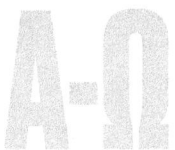

Master the light within as its observed in the 7 churches of the body; the 7 guiding spirits quickening the way to 'Throne of Grace'; and as its reflected in the planetary pantheon, focal points of other dimensions observable in this earth plane; audible as musical tones and seen in crystals, congealed light, which provide orderly vibrations which energetically assist particular to each of the body's centers.

SATURN

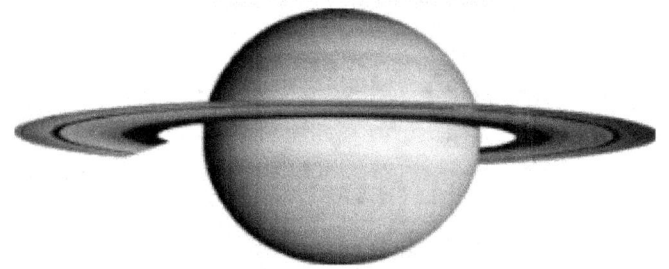

THE FIRST SEAL
EPHESUS—GONADS—DO (TONE)
RUBY—0 DIMENSIONS

PLANETARY ◇ PANTHEON

THE FIRST SEAL—EPHESUS—GONADS—SATURN—DO(TONE)—RUBY—0 DIMENSIONS

Purify the forces and return to the original purpose. Regaining control brings about complete restoration of the law of healing and supply. Saturn teaches us to make the best of the changes that come our way, be it relationships, activities, associations, environments, that all change may be developmental through the choices we make with them, that they may become lessons in patience to temper these changes with a spiritual ideal of Union in God.

NEPTUNE

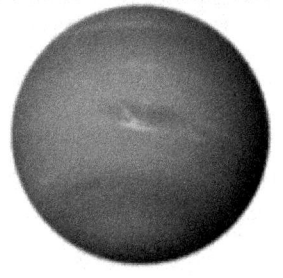

THE SECOND SEAL
SMYRNA—LYDIG TISSUE—RE (TONE)
CITRINE—MANY DIMENSIONS

PLANETARY PANTHEON

THE SECOND SEAL—SMYRNA— LYDIG—NEPTUNE—RE(TONE)— CITRINE—MANY DIMENSIONS

The regenerating wheel opens the center, where pure energy rises from the gonads to create mental forms and concepts. Regaining control will mean no regression from partial regeneration. Neptune teaches us to use a quick perception and intuition for mental and spiritual development, and to bring with it peace, harmony, and a more joyous perception. It reveals an urge for excitement, giving attraction to large bodies of water and an affinity toward the mystical, and teaching of the materializing influences of spirit and so inspires worship of the heroic.

MARS

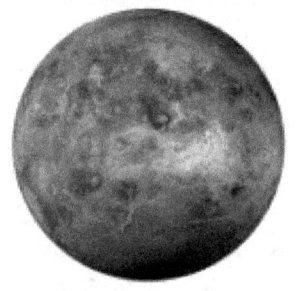

THE THIRD SEAL
PERGAMOS—ADRENAL GLAND—MI (TONE)
TOPAZ—I DIMENSION

PLANETARY ✡ PANTHEON

THE THIRD SEAL—PERGAMOS— ADRENAL—MARS—MI(TONE)— TOPAZ—1 DIMENSION

The major source of physical energy, capable of stimulating the body into action; with self control one can release the hormones from the adrenal into the bloodstream and directly cleanse all old patterns of energy and regenerating self at will. Mars teaches us to direct our energies with an ideal that we may judge and keep pure to this ideal our motives, so as to not lead to madness, anger, or a hard-headedness, that they not become expressions of animosity and covetousness, but are instead tempered and so teach patience, understanding, grace, and mercy.

VENUS

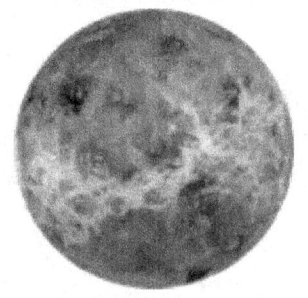

THE FOURTH SEAL
THYATIRA—THYMUS GLAND—FA (TONE)
EMERALD—4 DIMENSIONS

PLANETARY ✡ PANTHEON

THE FOURTH SEAL—THYATIRA—THYMUS—VENUS—FA(TONE)—EMERALD—4 DIMENSIONS

Absolute control will be given to that person over all parts and functioning's of the body; a return to the first condition of consciousness; a complete mastery of environment when one remains true to that perfect pattern and purifies against the forces for personal satisfaction. Venus teaches us to express the motivation force of Love and to appreciate all its effects of beauty, art, the home, and all the influences which bring about the bright and cheerful. Through Venus comes the desire for lovely things, conditions, and experiences; this includes a love for the harmonious, romance, and that which makes for an artistic temperament.

URANUS

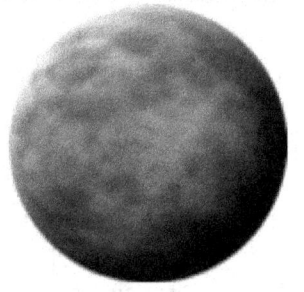

THE FIFTH SEAL
SARDIS—THYROID GLAND—SO (TONE)
SAPPHIRE—8 DIMENSIONS

PLANETARY ✦ PANTHEON

THE FIFTH SEAL—SARDIS—THYROID—URANUS—SO(TONE)—SAPPHIRE—8 DIMENSIONS

Opening of the thyroid center releases latent powers of the will. Overcoming this temptation will grant perpetual access to the creative forces. Uranus teaches us of the extremes in action and relationships, and to make practical experiences and applications of the interest in the mystical; to set ideals in the spiritual forces and keep busy; to find our spiritual ideal in Christ and keep active; to evaluate routines and be ever mindful of them.

JUPITER

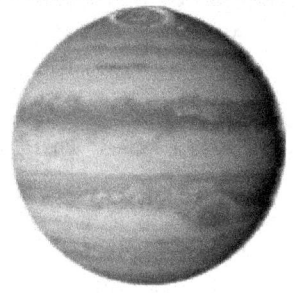

THE SIXTH SEAL
PHILADELPHIA—PINEAL GLAND—LA (TONE)
AMETHYST—5 DIMENSIONS

PLANETARY ✡ PANTHEON

THE SIXTH SEAL—PHILADELPHIA— PINEAL—JUPITER—LA(TONE)— AMETHYST—5 DIMENSIONS

The cosmic seat of memory which records all experiences and compares them with the perfect pattern within the soul, the ruling force of the Christ Consciousness. Jupiter teaches us to see all as whole and to apply this consciousness towards leadership of the masses. Jupiter teaches us to be cooperative, loving, helpful, and protective; to be soft-hearted, strong, mighty, and powerful; to be benevolent and urge others on.

MERCURY

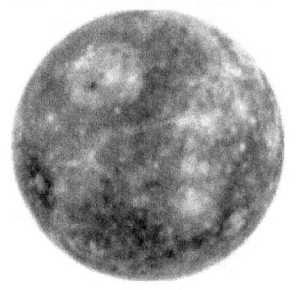

THE SEVENTH SEAL
LAODICEA—PITUITARY GLAND—TI (TONE)
DIAMOND—7 DIMENSIONS

PLANETARY PANTHEON

THE SEVENTH SEAL—LAODICEA—PITUITARY—MERCURY—TI(TONE)—DIAMOND—7 DIMENSIONS

The sounding of the 7 angels reflects purification and the pituitary gland as the regulatory gland of the entire body. Be only satisfied with this highest and master gland in control. It is the union of personality and the superconscious; the combined will of God and will of man flowing from a point at which man merges with the Divine. It releases energy that nourishes the system for healing and supply. Mercury teaches us to direct our thought to think through our problems and find answers; a sense of reasoning, good judgement, and sense of justice. Through Mercury we are attracted to problems not solved by others, and are innately students with great visions and mental acuteness that brings the knowledge to give oneself power to glorify God and honor our selected purposes in life. It is the indissoluble union.

Hear, oh Israel the lord thy God is One...
-Deuteronomy 6:4-5

THERE IS ONLY ONENESS. INTEGRATE INTO THIS AWARENESS, FOR WE ARE ALL CORPUSCLE OF THE ONE GOD. INTEGRATE, ALIGN, BE WHOLE. LET THIS MIND BE IN YOU WHICH WAS ALSO IN CHRIST JESUS

Reason this within you which Jesus Christ also reasoned, Who, being in the form of God, did not consider it robbery to be equal with God: But made himself of no reputation and took upon himself the form of a servant, and was in the likeness of men: And, being found in fashion as a man, he humbled himself, and became obedient to death, even the death of the cross. Wherefore God also has highly exalted him, and given him a name which is above every name; That at the name of Jesus every knee should bow, of those in heaven, of those on earth, and those under the earth, And every tongue shall confess that Jesus Christ is the LORD, to the glory of God his Father..

   -Philippians 2:5-11

Just keep the law. The law is love. Love is God, and our conduct is a ritual of attunement. When we die to ourselves and glorify the savior; when we manifest the fruits of the spirit toward others and awaken the divine within, we attune to the source of all force and grow into the dignity of Godhood—One with all, One with God.

HE THAT WILL BE GREATEST AMONG YOU WILL BE SERVANT TO ALL

Renew yourself in spirit seek the company of angels. The 'New Jerusalem' isn't as a place alone, but as a condition, an experience of the soul, an unfolding of self as Christ. Quicken this through prayer, talking to God, and meditation, listening to God. God is, and he rewards those who diligently seek him.

YOU ARE SONS OF GOD, SO ACT LIKE IT. HONOR YOUR SOUL AS CHRIST TEACHES. INSPIRE ALL WITH THE POWER THAT FLOWS THROUGH YOU AND BE LIFTED UP WITH GREATER ABILITIES TO REACH MORE.

Our Father in heaven, hallowed be thy name. Thy kingdom come. Thy will be done, as in heaven so on earth. Give us bread for our needs from day to day. And forgive us our offences, as we have forgiven our offenders; And do not let us enter into temptation, but deliver us from error. Because thine is the kingdom and the power and the glory for ever and ever. Amen.

   -Matthew 6:9-13

EVERYDAY MAKE OF LIFE A RITUAL TO GLORIFY GOD, THE SOURCE OF ALL FORCE, AND HONOR SELF, HIS TEMPLE

The body is the temple of the living God — Spirit is the life and mind - its builder; keep a mental image thats cooperative with the energies of the physical body.

Fill your mind and being with the expectancy of God that the body and mind may be constituted more perfectly for the manifestations of His forces.

Meditate, pray, and fast. Quicken the Spirit and Be whole; move the energy up from your sacral, direct and straight up to the crown; let flow the light of life through your eye of life and back flow grace through all your body. Accomplish this with service to the one god.

SIT COMFORTABLY ERECT AND RELAXED

Surround yourself with the protection of Christ's Light - be wholly the Light. Consider your power as you balance in equanimity and compose yourself in magnanimity.

PRAYER

God is the source of all force. You needn't worry when you can pray. Call on God and live by faith. Draw close to God and he will draw close to you. Pray:

Thy will O God; not mine, but Thine, be done in me, through me. Lord, here I am, use me, send me where I am needed.

NECK EXERCISES

Tilt head forward, backward, and to each side — making sure not to shrug or strain. Do this 3 times for each side. Tilt head forward and rotate clockwise and then counter-clockwise. Do this 3 times for both directions.

BREATH WORK

Breath Is the basis for the living organism.

Breathe a deep diaphragmatic breath; then breathe into the chest cavity; then lift and draw your shoulders back; after a moment's hold exhale in reverse order. Repeat this three times.

Next, place a finger to the side of your left nostril and hold closed; draw air though the right nostril and exhale through the mouth; close the right nostril and draw air through the left nostril and exhale through the right nostril.

CHANTING

The angels sing that God's glory be manifest. So to seek in all earnestness to make God conscious of you. Quicken the spirit. Chant:

'Yah—hay—vah—hay'

'Ahrrr—eee—ohmmm'

FOCUS, THINK, AND FEEL INTO YOUR AFFIRMATION OF UNION

The kingdom of heaven is within. Turn within to see if you are being true to yourself; know yourself, it is the ultimate revelation.

Ask without hidden motive and be surrounded by your answer. Be enveloped by what you desire, that your gladness be full.
-Nag Hammadi John 16:~24

BASK IN THE GLORY OF GOD

Be still and know that I am God.
-Psalms 46:10

BE
THAT
WHICH
YOU
PRAY
FOR

ENLIGHTENED ATHLETICS DIETARY PROTOCOL

3X WEEK

WHITE POTATO SKINS

DAIRY PRODUCTS

20%

BREAD:
RYE, WHOLE WHEAT,
PUMPERNICKEL

80%

FRUIT
OLIVE OIL
SPROUTED ALMONDS
WATER
FRESH VEGETABLES:
2-3 ABOVE GROUND VEGETABLES -
TO-
1 BELOW GROUND VEGETABLE

DRIED BEANS

DESSERT

CRACKERS
RICE

MEAT:
FISH, FOUL, LAMB

SOUP

EGG YOLKS

COFFEE OR TEA (W/OUT MILK)

NUTS AND
NUT BUTTER

SWEETENERS:
BEET SUGAR, RAW HONEY,
MAPLE SYRUP

G L O R I F Y   G O D
H O N O R   S E L F

Coordinate the 3rd Cervical, 9th Dorsal, and 4th Lumbar centers to effect a spiritual distribution through the 7 centers of the body:

Vibrational therapy (provided in consultation) - to equalize the extremities circulation as related to nerve impulses, and to assist nerves to feel out their roots through the system for the activity of impulse and to work with and coordinate with another. It attunes the vibration of the body to gold and silver - adding to or taking from impulses within the system from which those senses react in the brain itself.

Regulatory form of osteopathic therapy for structural correction and autonomic (sympathetic) coordination where the cerebrospinal and sympathetic nervous systems form conjunctions which produce coordination and drainage in the system.

Ensure there is a real desire to spiritually quicken, a willingness to be persistent, consistent, and patient. Patience as an active positive awareness of self and the continuity of life. Practice of patience is the basis of the virtues. It begets hope, faith, and makes for growth.

There must be an integration of heart, of mind, of purpose, of intent; a daily application of spiritual truth for the benefit of those in contact.

HEALTH FUNDAMENTALS

As the divine within is touched and awakened the body is healed.

Earthing - keep in the open, outside, and close to earth

Exercise - counteract the daily routine, especially by walking during evening

Eliminations - keep normal and proper eliminations, and make use of colonics

Sleep - ensure 6-7 hours of sleep per night, if stressed sleep 10-12 hours

Relax - make time to relax that you don't overtax the body

Masticate - chew your food thoroughly that you may enjoy it more and by activity of the glands in mouth and salivary glands keep the throat and bronchi healthier

Purify with food - eat plenty of lettuce that you may purify against those influences which attack the bloodstream

REJUVENATION FUNDAMENTALS

Fill your mind and being with the expectancy of God. There is no death, save in consciousness, so maintain an optimistic outlook about the body's potential for longevity, for aging continues only until one does what one knows to do, and the leaves undone what one knows not to do.

There is a creative power of our attitudes in shaping the physical body, so see what you eat doing what you would have it do, for what we eat and what we think, especially when taken together, make us what we are.

Rejuvenation Toolkit:
Enlightened Athletics Dietary Protocol; Nascent iodine; Enema (and colonic); Castor oil (Palma Christi) Hot Pack; Consume Olive oil (3-5 teaspoons per day); Eat a few sprouted almonds per day; Epsom salt bath with oil of Pine needles; Proper hydration (I gallon daily); Glass of warm lemon water upon rising; Salsify (oyster plant); Triphala; Monoatomic Gold

Massage (peanut oil or olive oil - alternate daily)
Massage Rationale: Inactivity causes many of those portions along the spine from which impulses are received to the various organs to be lax, or taut, or to allow some to receive greater impulse than others. The massage aids the ganglia to receive impulse from nerve forces as it aids circulation through the various portions of the organism.

3 DAY APPLE FAST

Purge the body of toxic accumulations with this simple and easy to follow fast, consuming sheep-noise variety apples for three days.
Ensure the apples are thoroughly washed, raw and unpeeled.
Drink only warm water throughout the 3 day fast, and upon the fourth day consume 2 tablespoons of olive oil in the morning and follow with the Enlightened Athletics Dietary Protocol. This detox will purify the system; improving assimilation and elimination, and be almost euphoric in effect.

Resulting from a weakened esophageal sphincter that allows gastric juices to damage mucosa of esophagus. The problem isn't isolated however, and is systemic, and is either resulting from an infection of a chronic nature with an effect on the liver, pancreas, and spleen; or has its causative factor in an autonomic nervous system malfunction in the mid dorsal region from D4 to D9 which effects the liver or directly effects the stomach when digestion starts. Improper function of the liver, pancreas, and spleen effectually suppresses assimilation in the lacteal duct area of the small intestine, the Peyers patch, making a tendency for the condition to perpetuate itself.

Therapy:
•Enlightened Athletics Dietary Protocol with sprouted almonds and a daily sip of olive oil
•Colonic irrigation (cycling with 3 on the first month; 1 on the second month; 2 on the third; and 1 on the fourth)
•Osteopathic manipulation to the mid dorsal region
•Saffron Tea before every meal, unless eating only raw vegetables (3tsp of Yellow Saffron in 16oz - steeped for 30 minutes)
•1 tsp of Milk Magnesia after every meal
•Drink large quantities of Elm Water (add a pinch of powdered elm to water with ice and let to steep for 3 minutes)

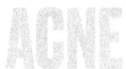

ACNE

Acne, occurring principally through unbalanced eliminations in the liver and kidneys, and in turn expressed in the clogging of superficial capillaries and small lymphatic vessels, has multiple factors which can be identified and addressed as follows:

•Improper diet at beginning of menses - correct with Enlightened Athletics High Performance Institute Diet (+ no bananas, strawberries, or raw apples).

•Glandular reactions and gradual building of difficulty is related to the glands and circulation - correct by cleansing glands - 1 tablespoon of Sulphur, 1 tablespoon of Rochelle salts, 1 tablespoon of Cream of Tartar (mix thoroughly and enjoy 1 tsp before breakfast). Use of nascent iodine also advised.

•Circulatory problems, often brought about by a back injury, however mild, can be resolved easily with regular osteopathic adjustment and massage with great effect to skin appearance.

•Local therapy - cleanse thoroughly with soap, not picking at adhesion, but applying ice cube in cloth to freeze affected areas for 2-5 minutes.

ALLERGIES

An allergy refers to a hypersensitive state due to exposure to a particular allergen (immediate or delayed) including: serum sickness, allergic drug reactions contact dermatitis, anaphylactic shock; usually manifested in the gastrointestinal tract, the skin and the respiratory tract.

Common primary causes:
Poor circulation; inadequate eliminations; acid/ alkaline imbalance

Therapy:
•Chiropractic adjustment
•Enlightened Athletics dietary protocol
•Hydrotherapy colonic or enema

Local therapy:
•Herbal breathing inhalant

ALZHEIMERS

The nervous system and brain are dependent upon the rest of the body for removal of wastes and supply of nutrients. Assimilation and Elimination are key in both understanding of cause and for designation of therapy. Therapies designed to cleanse and nurture the tissues of the brain:

•Spiritually: Foster patience. It is the basis and most beautiful of the virtues.
•Mentally: naturalistic subjugative hypnosis
•Physically: Spinal manipulations, followed by massage and a vibrational device to stimulate the nervous system (provided in consult)

AMYOTROPHIC LATERAL SCLEROSIS

Often originating with a karmic etiology, with that first cell introduced in the body. This etiology is similar enough that the article on MS mav be found useful as well. The disease process begins with lack of assimilation. This then begets a deficiency of the substances in the bloodstream that would otherwise be carried throughout the system, and replenish and rebuild the nerve and muscle tissues affected. The process is gradual and can take ears to develop into a disease.

Therapy: Begin with a spiritual purpose and attitude change (Suggested Reading: Deuteronomy 30; Exodus 19:5)

•Enlightened Athletics Dietary Protocol (additionally, low carbs and no alcohol)

•Use of vibrational therapy device (provided in consult)

•Massage (following the use of the vibrational therapy device) 45 minutes from toes to head (including extremities) concentrating on the spine, especially the sciatic center, lumbar access, and brachial center.

•Every three days In the morning add a drop of each of the following solutions to half a glass of water: gold chloride solution - one grain per ounce of distilled water: bromide soda solution - 2 grains per ounce of distilled water.

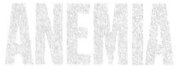

ANEMIA

When there exists a languidness only loosely associated with another defined illness, some degree of anemia is usually concomitant.

Brought about by multiple factors, including: decreased intake or assimilation of iodine, vitamins, or food; lymphatic condition; glandular imbalance; or lung pathology.

Common specific etiologic factors include: malfunctioning thyroid; faulty eliminations; incoordination of adrenal gland and lacteal area of Peers patches; catarrhal conditions in digestive tract.

Therapy:
•Enlightened Athletics dietary protocol (w/no shellfish)
•Regular colonics eliminations should be kept
•Osteopathic manipulations (especially the 7th dorsal to 2nd lumbar)
•Infrared therapy - 30 minutes/twice a week
•Nascent iodine course

Be mindful that bone marrow, which creates red blood cells, requires proper nutriment and arouse the normal activity from the system itself.

APHONIA

The loss of the ability to speak is most commonly due to an injury to the 2nd or 3rd dorsal causing coordinate dorsal ganglia patches to atrophy. Less common as a cause is toxic buildup from poor eliminations which leads to disassociation of larynx and throat from the rest of the body. Fear is a concomitant factor that creates lesions in patches with subsequent overflow impulse throughout body.

Therapy is to cleanse the system with specific reference to the hepatic circulation.

Therapy:
•Hydrotherapy colonic or enema
•Castor oil pack
•Epsom salt pack
•Gentle osteopathic manipulations series
•Enlightened Athletics dietary protocol modified to include lots of citrus juice
•Meditate daily upon the use of voice, mind, and actions being used in material, mental, spiritual aid to others.

Therapy of last resort:
•Formal hypnosis

ARTERIOSCLEROSIS

Direct the material, mental, and spiritual forces toward recuperation. As the divine within is touched and awakened, so too is the body healed.

Common to arteriosclerosis is the multiplicity of factors involved. When one abnormal function is aided and abetted by another, symptoms appear and pathology occurs. Keep in mind the various causes and symptoms manifested in the pathology that adjustment of the body may be made more logical and complete; that the application, physically, mentally, materially to those things that would bring a better balance, including all effects and causes, are to be taken into consideration. The disturbances, usually being of a deep-seated nature, require a great deal of change in the mental attitude, metal outlook, else applications are only helpful experiences for the activities being carried on. Balance the body forces:

•Osteopathic Adjustments: towards lumbosacral area, mid dorsal, upper dorsal (2nd, 3rd, 4th)

•Enlightened Athletics Dietary Protocol (+ no red meat; little starch or sugar; lots of vitamin B1, as found in yellow foods; lots of green foods)

•Regular Massage: Balance neurological impulse along spine. 2 oz. olive oil (heated); 2 oz. tincture of myrrh; 10 drops of calamus oil.

•Regular Colonics and Hydrotherapy

•Outdoor exercise, especially walking.

ARTHRITIS

Chiefly concerning Arthritis of calcium buildup (senescent; hypertrophic; osteopathic), and not involving inflammation.

Etiology: poor eliminations; inadequate assimilations; lack of iodine; chemical imbalance; lack of proper distribution of energies.

Therapy:

•Correct the assimilations: control digestive abnormalities

•Increase eliminations; castor oil packs; various eliminants; colonics; enemas; hot baths; epsom salt baths; fume baths

•Improve the nerve supply to the muscles and tendons and the affected organs through massaging Peanut Oil and Olive Oil (alternating each day) after hot bath.

•Enlightened Athletics Dietary Protocol; add gelatin to recipes for optimal use of vitamins with raw vegetables: watercress, chard, mustard greens, kale, carrots, celery, Romain lettuce, beet tops, raw nuts, especially sprouted almonds and filberts, vegetable and citrus juices.

Cooked vegetables especially salsify, parsnips, potato peelings from baked potato (not the mass), Jerusalem artichoke (at least once a week cooked and raw), Black bread (rye, pumpernickel, etc.)

•avoid red and fried meat, pork, carbonated water, alcohol, apples, bananas, strawberries, tomatoes, cabbage, starchy foods, and stimulants

BALDNESS AND HAIR COLOR

Listen to the body, for baldness isn't just a sign of aging, but of a glandular deficiency as either the primary or contributing cause of the condition with a subluxation of the spine another equally common primary cause.

Cure baldness and restore hair color by restoring thyroid secretions affecting circulation; through osteopathic manipulation; E.A Dietary Protocol; and local application.

Therapy:

•Enlightened Athletics Dietary Protocol, adding potato skins (not pulp), carrots, and three seafood meals per week, citrus juices; Nascent iodine or herbal tonic (provided in consultation) .

•Avoid Fried, greasy foods, fried meats, starches, refined sugars, onion, and garlic.

•Massage: l tsp. Pure crude oil to scalp (keep on for 45 min); cleanse with 20% grain alcohol (vodka); follow this with vaseline scalp massage.

•Violet light treatment on scalp, spine, scapula, and umbilical area for a total of 10 minutes daily.

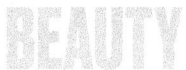
BEAUTY

Be free of any blemish of any nature.
Keep a spiritual goal and ideal, something beyond one's self — give of self
Keep a healthy state of mind, an equilibrium and correct flow of glandular secretion, that the hormones released are of a healthy and beautiful nature. For as the body is built it thinks, and as it thinks the body is built — as within, so without.
Therapy:
•Enlightened Athletics Dietary Protocol.
•Thoroughly massage for at least 20 minutes one of the following emollients a day, alternating which each day: olive oil, for it stimulates muscular and mucus membrane activity; olive oil with Myrrh, for it is carried into the pores toward folds or scars in the tissue for coagulation (heat the olive oil first and add an equal portion of myrrh, making just enough for each day); camphorated oil, as it produces soothing and stimulation, and when combined with the others will make for a new skin.

BLINDNESS

Losing sight mandates the facing of self.
Congestion of visual apparatus; light and sensation deflected due to lesions in centers along and outside the spinal cord, generally from the first and fourth dorsal to the first cervical. This is where the cerebrospinal and sympathetic nervous systems make contact, an intersection with mental-emotional and psychic energies, and thus therapy is both physical and psychological. Additional or alternative pathologies include: a greater requirement of the assimilation of gold to supply reflex necessary in nerve plasm for the healing of nerve tissue; Impingement of nerves that govern eyesight, circulation then cut off and affecting optic nerve to carry sensation for sight to the brain.
Therapy:
•Keep an encouraging environment, and make the time to meditate and pray often.
•Pray 'Let Thine will be done, in me and through me' Meditate to Know Thyself and awaken more the vision from within. Be pleasing in the Living God's sight. It is the purpose for which each soul enters earth. Accept in soul and purpose a Universal Christ Consciousness. It is the purest vibration for healing. Grow into the changes, and with patience, persistence, and consistency use what is obtained in a better manner.
•Enlightened Athletics' 'Dietary Protocol
•Gentle Osteopathic manipulation
•Colonics, fume baths, and gentle laxatives
•Vibratory Devices (available in consult)

BREAST CANCER

Attitude - what will you do with life if you recover? Awareness of, and attunement to, higher ideals and healing forces is of major importance. Lead emphasis be placed on a prayerful and purposeful state of mind.
Therapy:
•Enlightened athletics dietary protocol, adding, and continue with after recovery, sprouted almonds), cooked asparagus
Avoid meat
•Take five glycothymoline drops by mouth three times daily. Prepare fruits and vegetables with gelatin.
•Nascent iodine to promote glandular eliminations.
•Castor oil packs to promote assimilative function.
•Massage affected area massage around the affected breast with cocoa butter to stimulate drainage and lymphatic activity.

BURSITIS

In breaking up congestions and expelling the accumulations about the bursa, one will need to focus on improving circulation and on increasing eliminations until there is no further mucus indicated near the colon area.

Therapy:
- Regular colonic hydrotherapy and senna laxatives
- Apply warm epsom salt packs whenever /wherever there are pains or accumulations
- Regular oil massages
- Regular sauna
- 5 days on/off of gold cocktail to supply nerve energy - made by separately mixing 1 grain gold chloride in 1 ounce water and 2 grains bromide of soda in 1 ounce water; place one drop of the gold solution and two drops of the soda solution in half a glass of water and drink immediately.

BUST SIZE

Women which desire a larger bust can with the following therapies safely and naturally lift and increase bust size.
Therapy:
Massage:
•Massage cocoa butter under the arm (arm pit area); below the breast; and between them. With persistency one can increase them to whatever size one likes.
•Stretching and expanding chest frame exercises to be increased gradually, without strain:
-Arm circles
-Push-pulls

In order to decrease bust one merely has to instead of massaging the gland around the breast tissue massage the breast tissue itself with cocoa butter.

CATARACTS

To overcome cataracts requires improved circulation and elimination, that the accumulations in the sensory system may be eliminated.

Less common causes are: spinal lesions, digestive disturbances, dietary insufficiency, mental attitude, mechanical injury, and constitutional condition.

Therapy should be approached on all levels - spiritual, mental, and physical. The body must be convinced within self, else little healing will be had with the physical applications.

Therapy:
•Osteopathic adjustment - C1, C2, C3, D1, D2, D3
•Massage with peanut oil - Emphasis to spine, mastoid, temple, and chin (2x/day)
•Spiritual Counseling (prayer and meditation)

CHRONIC FATIGUE

In overcoming Chronic Fatigue there is broad systemic involvement, but most usually originating with poor eliminations, and so a variety of therapies are used in concert to achieve a holistic effect.

Therapy:
- Enlightened Athletics Dietary Protocol
- Proper hydration with pure water
- Regular hydrotherapy colonics and senna laxatives
- Castor oil packs
- Regular and rigorous exercise
- Osteopathic manipulation (or Vibratory massage) with subsequent massage to remove any subluxations or pressures on nerves and regulate sympathetic nervous system
- Specific electro-therapy device (provided in consultation) to balance circulation
- Nascent iodine to stimulate and purify the glandular system
- Build the body for God's service, that the body and mind may be constituted more perfectly for the manifestations of God.

COLD

Keep the body alkaline - keep alkalized. A cold develops in the presence of an acid condition. Add a teaspoon of baking soda to each glass of water. Release all resentments and anger - forgive it all away. The glands secrete poisons when angry. Instead of resentments, Love. Rest to balance the function of the autonomic nervous system.

Therapy:
•Consume extra Citrus fruit
•Keep a mostly liquid diet
•Chew excessively all food
•Occasional tsp of Rye whiskey
•Senna laxative or Enema
•Abhyanga (massage) with olive oil
-Massage Rationale: Inactivity causes many of those portions along the spine from which impulses are received to the various organs to be lax, or taut, or to allow some to receive greater impulse than others. The massage aids the ganglia to receive impulse from nerve forces as it aids circulation through the various portions of the organism.

COLITIS

Preceded by a cold or intestinal flu and sometimes by an injury, colitis always occurs with lymphatic disturbance and inflammation throughout the intestinal wall. Because of this lymph can become toxic to the entire body, especially the liver, and because of the toxic effect on Peyers patches, the lacteal ducts that are closely related to the assimilatory process are hindered and food can no longer be made to rebuild the body tissues, hence a tenseness in replenishing and tendency towards anemia.

Therapy directed at restoring proper function of lymph through rest; eliminating the inflammatory process; balancing the PH by soothing the lymphatic activity; and coordinating the nervous system.

Therapy:
•Enlightened Athletics Dietary Protocol (additionally incorporate tuberous vegetables; no meats (only fish and fowl); no fried foods; eat strength giving foods, especially a great deal of fruit and juices, especially citrus juices; Prunes;
pineapple; refrain from pastries and sweets.
•Wild Ginseng Fusion
•Beef Juice - 2 tbsps day
•Concorde grape poultice layered on abdomen

COLOR BLINDNESS

Direct the material, mental, and spiritual forces toward recuperation.

Technically resulting from nerve energies deflected from origin in 2nd, 3rd, and 4th dorsal sympathetic ganglia, these coordinating through vagus nerve in 3rd, 4th, and 5th cervical ganglia; and observed as insufficient nerve impulse in lower cervical optic enters for replenishing of the eyes and carrying away refuse. One must correct the condition in the dorsal area to then stimulate more the cervical area to supply the rebuilding of nerve forces.

Therapy:
•Enlightened Athletics Dietary Protocol
•Osteopathic Adjustment to the dorsal area - correcting the 2nd, 3rd, and 4th segments (3 per week × 3 weeks, or until dorsal is perfectly aligned - as seen by the balance of circulation between the left and right temple), only afterward beginning on the cervical.

As the divine within is touched and awakened, so too is the body healed.

CONSTIPATION

Most commonly constipation has it's origin in and acidity created in the assimilating system of the body. Subluxations and an acid reacting diet also causal though less common

Constipation can be considered as intestinal indigestion where there is expressed a packing of fecal material in the large bowel. Brought on by negative manifestations of the adrenal gland which bring acidity in the stomach and duodenal area, it translates into decreased function of lymph, and reabsorption of intestinal wastes.

Therapy:
•Enlightened Athletics Dietary Protocol
•Osteopathic Adjustment Series
•Intestinal Cleansing - Colonics, Enemas, and Eliminants
•Castor Oil Pack
•Abdominal Massage with Olive Oil

Keep assimilations and eliminations normal. The assimilations build the body and will aid in resuscitating it so long as eliminations are good.

CROHNS

The most common cause is viral, an intestinal flu that settles in the intestines and disturbs the lymphatics. Alternatively, it can come about by intestinal inflammation further up the digestive system, or directly caused by pressures on the spinal nerves which govern the digestive system.

Therapy:
•Enlightened Athletics Dietary Protocol (Modified w/ focus on consuming grapes)
•Hydrotherapy colonic
•Osteopathic Manipulation
•Herbal Formula of: Ginseng, Ginger, Lactated Pepsin, Stillingia
•Grape Poultice on Abdomen

Pray for and expect healing

CEREBROVASCULAR ACCIDENT

There must be a real desire to regain good health and willingness to be persistent, consistent, and patient in achieving it.

The functioning of the extremities and what are called the locomotor faculties are not entirely dependent upon the brain. If balance between the circulatory, sympathetic, and locomotive centers are brought back to a balance full function can be restored.

Therapies aimed to: Prevent circulation from progressing to a more toxic condition; Eliminate poisons; Remove pressures on sympathetic and locomotory centers; Aid the body to rebuild

Therapy:
- Enlightened Athletics Dietary Protocol (modifying to eat lightly)
- Enemas - beginning with three on the first day and daily thereafter
- Osteopathic treatment - gently first and more vigorous progressively
- Hot Epsom salt packs
- Massage spine and extremities (massage away from head toward extremities)

DIABETES

Primary physiological consideration is a malfunction in the pancreas gland with ramifications that extend through coordination with the liver. There is a tendency in the pancreas in diabetes type 1 and 2 to create too much sugar and handle carbohydrates in such a way that form an excess of sugar.

Causation linked to disturbance in cerebrospinal centers: 6th, 7th, 8th, and 9th dorsal sympathetic ganglia. These give impulse to the liver and pancreas primarily, as well as the spleen, that brings an imbalance through the pancreas and the circulation and the coordination between the liver and pancreas, thus causing glycosuria - diabetes.

In appraising the need for therapy, osteopathic or chiropractic manipulation will not always be necessary, but will certainly always be useful.

Dietary correction is highly useful and has more to do with the helpful reactions in therapy than any other application.

Therapy:
•Osteopathic manipulation
•Enlightened Athletics Dietary Protocol with Jerusalem artichokes 3 to 6 times weekly (alternate between cooked and raw);
plenty of fruits, especially apples; leafy vegetables;
Little coffee or tea and without cream or sugar; no carbonated beverages or alcohol

DIVERTICULITIS

There are several factors in the genesis of diverticular disease of the colon, a pouch like out-pocketing consisting of mucosa and serosal layers. These can be sourced back to lesions occurring after abdominal surgery or poor eliminations resulting as dyssynergy of autonomic nervous system.

Therapy:
•Castor oil pack for 4 hours every day, and half a teaspoon of Olive taken every two hours of treatment.
•Colonic - two per week after 3rd day of castor oil pack
•Senna laxative to maintain regularity
•Enlightened Athletics Dietary Protocol w/ primarily liquids and semisolid food for first two weeks.
•Massage body with emphasis along the spine with peanut oil and olive oil, daily alternating
•Nascent Iodine

DREAMS

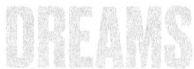

As we sleep we connect with the unconscious mind.

Find the theme of the action in your dream, the verbs of the narrative; see the action, then see the symbols; then begin to see the mirror of waking life. This is the dreamers way of being.

If you will attune your awareness to those metaphors packaged for your conscious mind you will grow into a superconscious state. When you leverage this time for your conscious unfoldment into higher consciousness you will lead the dreamers way of being.

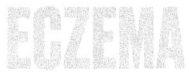

ECZEMA

Therapy:
- Enlightened Athletics Dietary Protocol; modified to consume primarily vegetables, especially carrots, okra, squash, and fruits - though sparingly
- Avoid raw apples and bananas
- Avoid all fried foods, carbonated drinks, candy, sugar, pastries, potatoes, white bread, pork, beef, butter, greases, and fats
- Drink Mullein Tea every evening (let steep for 30 minutes)

EPILEPSY

Where epilepsy is a primary pathophysiological concern there will be found a cold spot felt on the abdomen which is an adhesion(s) and which is found between the lacteal ducts and the caecum. It is often due to a reflex action from an initial injury to a spinal segment, particularly in the sacral-coccygeal region. Also often, it may due to a trauma on the upper right quadrant of the abdomen or in the region of the umbilicus during or after birth. Less often, its due to a post natal infection of the umbilical area. Also, but least often, sometimes adrenals and gonads have reflex action via autonomic nervous system on the pineal and pituitary glands.

Therapy to address the incoordination produced in cerebrospinal nervous system and autonomic nervous system; with reciprocal action in Lacteal ducts and spinal lesions:

•3-day series of Castor Oil Packs (these are preliminary but have a reciprocal effect with Osteopathic manipulation)
•Osteopathic manipulations especially where relevant nerve plexus is affected
•Massage with peanut oil and/or olive oil to break up lesions and adhesions
•Couple teaspoons of olive oil before bed (Oil absorbs through lacteal ducts and helps increase flow through them)

FLU

3 types of flu: A- known as a biannual epidemic; B- sporadic in nature: C- very mild.
The principal sites involved are the respiratory tract and gastrointestinal tract. Sufficient hemoglobin of proper functioning and white blood cell swill make for immunity and overcoming of the flu.

Causes: cold and congestion causes for which are often over-acidity and mechanical pressure on the cerebrospinal system); poor
eliminations; deficiencies in the blood supply (humoral and/or cellular); poor diet; or combination.

Therapy is to address underlying issue before symptoms:
•laxatives (senna-based)
•massages
•osteopathic manipulations;
•hydrotherapy (for severe disturbances)
•Enlightened Athletics dietary protocol
•Rectified bicarbonate or Alka Seltzer.
•Consume 3 tablespoons per day of expectorant:
Egg white mixed with juice of I lemon, and, added slowly, I tbsp of honey, with 2 drops of glycerine added last

FRACTURES AND SPRAINS

Healing will come about as manifestation of spirit with the balance of the physical and mental body. The coagulation of electrical energies into tissue - callus formation - requires coordination of the body-whole with the proper eliminations of refuse energies as well as a balance of the sympathetic ganglia through adjustments and manipulations.

Therapy:
•General osteopathic manipulation and subsequent massage for better drainage

•Local massages alternating daily with the following: Heated olive oil and tincture of myrrh (equal parts); and salt soaked in apple vinegar

GOUT

A condition of arthritis, but distinct from other classifications, may be arrested and in time dissolved.

Cleanse the system with that regiment found in for Arthritis and renew the affected area with the following local therapy

Place over the affected area a cloth soaked in castor oil, a thin piece of plastic above it, and a hot pack for 30 mins - 1 hour on top. Afterward, cleanse the area with baking soda. Repeat daily.

HEADACHES

The nervous system, the digestive system and the circulatory system are all closely interrelated in the pathogenesis of headaches.
Common etiology is related to pressure on nerve plexus opposite of the pneumogastric center, which reflexively transmits pressure to the brain as a headache. This is primarily due to inadequate eliminations.

Therapy:
•Colonic to resolve intestinal abnormalities and malfunctions.
•Proper hydration, senna laxatives, and enemas also advised.
•Osteopathic manipulation and massage to resolve another common etiology of subluxation in spine.
•Alkalize the body - Enlightened Athletics Dietary Protocol
•Dissolve emotional and mental stress by fixing the attitude be kind and helpful to others.

HEMOPHILIA

Hemophilia is a deficiency due to improper assimilation of the elements which are necessary to build vital energies in the glands, and their functions in the body, including proper coagulation of blood and ability to build walls of blood vessels.

This deep-seated, but correctable ailment can be inherited or developed. The defects might be removed by a process involving a vibratory device provided in consultation. This will constructively effect the lacteal duct center, the largest Peyers patch, an area important for control of assimilation which also indirectly controls circulation.

Therapy is to return the body to normal function:

Consistent application of vibratory device (provided) which makes for proper glandular activity, not adding or attempting to make the chemical reactions but providing the substrate for better activity in coordination of glands, organs, and lacteal duct.

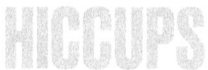

HICCUPS

A hiccup (hiccough) is the convulsion in the diaphragm where the esophagus enters the upper portion of the stomach.

Inhalant Therapy:
Inhalant to be made using bottle, cork, air tube and inhalant tube. Inhaling through each nostril 3 times 3 times a day, if necessary.
Recipe:
4 oz. good rye whiskey
20 minims (or drops) eucalyptus oil
5 minims rectified turpentine oil
15 minims compound benzoin tincture
10 minims pine needle oil

HYPERTENSION

Most cases are due to an improper equilibrium of circulation - strain on the internal capillaries and emunctories. This leads to a plethoric condition in the veins and arteries which in turn effects the regulation of the circulation. Secondary etiology as lesions to spinal cord or nerve plexuses that control blood pressure or disturb hepatic circulation. Other causes are in the GI tract, Peyers Patches, or the circulatory system itself.

Emotional factors that mav be responsible include repression of anger and resentment, which affects the spleen and leads to hypertension.

Therapy promotes the equalization of circulation and stability of nerve forces.
•Get out of bed as soon as you wake up, eat half of a lemon, take a long walk, eat the other half of the lemon with a pinch of salt, drink as much water as possible; then lie down until completely relaxed before breakfast.
•Enlightened Athletics dietary protocol, plus extra bulbous vegetables and vegetable protein
•Hydrotherapy colonic
•Osteopathic adjustments
•Massage with peanut oil subsequent to adjustment

HYPOTHYROIDISM

Usually due to an imbalance of chemicals in the blood, and frequently also an excess of potassium and deficiency of iodine (which is essential for proper functioning of the thyroid gland)

Therapy:

- Vibrational treatments to regenerate and coordinate nervous systems
- Violet Light Therapy
- Enlightened athletics dietary protocol with emphasis on vegetables
- Osteopathic/Chiropractic manipulation
- Spinal massage with peanut and or olive oil
- Nascent iodine or thyroid extract
- Better attitude towards self and others

INTESTINAL CANCER

Poor eliminations, assimilations, over-acidity of the body are all contributing factors to intestinal cancers.

Therapies:
•Hydrotherapy colonic
•slippery elm or senna laxative
•castor oil enema
•1/8-1/4 grain of animated ash in glass of water/daily
•UV light treatment for 3 min 30 mins after drinking animated ash
•Castor oil/epsom salt packs along abdomen
•cold saffron tea
•Osteopathic manipulations (or use of vibrating massager along the spine)
•General massage

IODINE (NASCENT FORM)

A form of Iodine which has been electrified and liberated from its diatomic bond into a nascent state where it's paramagnetic charge carries energy throughout the body furnishing the element that's readily utilized for production of hormones (esp. T3 and T4) and detoxification of the body.

Though supplementing can help nearly every body, it's especially useful for those with iodine deficiency, which is to be expected when the prevalence of chlorine and fluorine ions in water supply is high, as halogens easily compete for iodine receptor sites.

KIDNEY DYSFUNCTION

Kidneys are as the negative pole of the body and focus of the lower hepatic circulation, while the liver is the positive pole and regulates the upper hepatic circulation. problems with either are usually reflected in the other.

Therapy:
•Enlightened Athletics Dietary Protocol adding Jerusalem Artichoke
•Lithia water
•Watermelon seed tea
•Osteopathic Therapy: to lower thoracic and lumbar (where nerve plexus are associated with kidney functioning
•Massage: on back location of kidneys w/ compound of mutton tallow, spirits of camphor, spirits of turpentine

Symptomatic Relief: hot packs of the following (separately): turpentine; mullein;
castor oil; glycothymoline; epsom salt

KIDNEY STONE

Observed as a physiological process instead of just had a condition of a stone in place, a kidney stone announces the process of precipitated or sedimented material - composed of a number of materials in the bloodstream by which the liquid excreted in the kidneys is saturated to such a degree that portions are no longer in solution and have begun the sedimentary or crystallization process. The overflow of toxins, which indicates an impaired liver and kidney, is carried and accumulated in the system without the proper flow in emunctory channels. Primary cause: Poor attitudes and emotions that cause destruction in the body. Intermediate cause: Incoordination in the eliminatory process.

Therapy:
Attitude shift for the increase of patience and persistence; meet experiences not in anger or wrath but in gentleness and the fruits of the spirit.

•Turpentine poultice
•General massage
•Osteopathic adjustment
•Enlightened Athletics Dietary Protocol - modification for easy assimilation: increase amount of cooked fruit and vegetables
•Mullein and watermelon seed teas
•Hydrotherapy colonic or enemas
•Castor oil pack

LARYNGITIS

The digestive tract, most typically being the seat of the problem, can be addressed with eliminants In order to correct the activity of the hepatic circulation by normalizing blood plasm in the division of blood supply and relieve the congestion of the liver.

Primary causative factors include usually either acute bacilli infection brought on by inhaling too much dirt and dust and/ or inadequate elimination. Therapies for both can be used in conjunction.

Therapy:
•Enlightened Athletics Dietary Protocol modified to consume citrus fruit juices and keep primarily a fruit/ veggie diet without white bread or meat
•Massage the 1st, 2nd, 3rd dorsal, cervical area, throat and chest
•Senna Tea and/or Senna Laxative
•Hydrotherapy colonic
•Turkish bath
•Dry sauna
•Inhalant made from:
1/2 tsp Benzoin tincture
1/2 tsp eucalyptus oil
Add to a pint of boiling water, breathe in fumes and place a towel over head

LEUKEMIA

The tissues of the body have their creation facilitated by hormones which coagulate the electrical forces into form. Globulins are acted upon by hormones released by glandular tissue which are activated by vitamins for the structural activity of the system.

Leukemia arises from being without proper activity of the structural portions of the body (especially through ribs, spleen, and pancreas with the digestive activities of the body). The whole process of the disease is caused by glandular disturbances from imbalanced chemical reactions in the body. This takes the form of an over abundance of white blood cells which then leads to a disruption of anabolic-catabolic balance of the body and a hardness of the lymph along the ribs and spine.

Biochemically, this is often resultant of an iodine deficiency, and sufficient Iodine is vital for the recovery from leukemia.

Therapy:
•Nutritionally - Fresh squeezed tree ripened orange juice
•Biochemically - Nascent Iodine regimen
•Osteopathically - Coordination of the spine
•Massage - especially D5, D6, D7

LUNG CANCER

Cancer is an entity unto itself that draws from the vitality of the body and represents a failure of natural processes of which may be caused by various forms of chronic irritation. Lung cancer caused by destructive bacilli in the blood or system.

Therapy:
•Hydrotherapy colonic
•Modified Enlightened Athletics Dietary Protocol and add small quantities of beef juice
•Rub iodex ointment mixed with animated ash over painful areas
•Every other day apply violet lamp or specialized UV lamp (provided in consult) over back opposite of lungs after consuming 1/8 grain of animated ash mixed with water
•2 minutes daily receive light emitted from shortwave mercury (or quartz) lamp at approximately 3ft away from the body
•Use of inhalant made from: rectified oil of turpentine, pine needle oil, eucalyptus oil, grain alcohol base

LUPUS

Primary Causative Factors are inadequate and incoordinate eliminations (defecation, urination, respiration, perspiration).
The object of therapy is to improve systemic functioning by improving elimination, assimilation, and circulation.

Therapy:
•Maintain an attitude of creative helpfulness and truly desire and expect to be healed
•Hydrotherapy colonics to clean intestines
•Enlightened Athletics Dietary Protocol
•Drink at least 8 glasses of water/day, Slippery Elm Bark Tea in morning, and American Yellow Saffron Tea in evening
•Osteopathic manipulation for systemic coordination
•Massage to clean hepatic organs
•Castor oil packs over abdomen to clear alimentary canal and stimulate liver
•Nascent iodine to purify glands

MENOPAUSE

Every woman can have a different menopausal experience depending primarily on the manner in which she faces life and her selected purpose for being here.

The body is capable of normal function, and change of the life situation can be met with equanimity. Often distresses experienced are due to pelvic organs and those of the eliminating system, as well as the upper hepatic circulation and the indeterminate reactions of impulses between the autonomic and cerebral spinal system.

To relieve headaches, hot/cold flashes, and irregularity of heart:
•Keep balanced and well rested
•Don't overstimulate the vital forces of the body, especially those related to the activities of reproduction
•Fast on oranges and lemons for five days, then half a tea cup of olive oil
•Epsom salt bath
•Olive oil massage
•Osteopathic manipulation
•Nascent iodine
•Calcium supplement

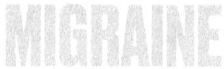

MIGRAINE

Most all migraines begin with congestion in the colon, a congestion often often preceded by a subluxation in the lumbar and sacral area, which then causes pressure on the sympathetic nerve centers and cerebrospinal system.

Therapy:
Applications should be made in a consistent and persistent manner; they may at first appear aggravating more than allaying.
•Colonic irrigation (enemas, hydrotherapy):
Cleanse sufficiently long enough for nutriment to be supplied into the colon's folds - two weeks apart, five times.
•1 hr of meditation a day for self-awareness and make sure to keep a helpful attitude - no complaining
•Osteopathic or chiropractic manipulation of the sixth and seventh dorsal, lower back, and lumbar axis.
•Enlightened Athletics Dietary Protocol with additional watercress, celery, lettuce, carrots, and prepare them with gelatin; remove sweets and chocolate

MOLES

Occuring in most, moles are a localized growth due to a glandular reaction and are best left alone from outer effect unless they cause a disturbance.

The following recipe should be applied and massaged around and over the mole twice a day for two hours with a two-day rest.

•Small amount of castor oil with a little amount of baking soda (only that necessary for massage of affected area) after massage the affected area will be sore for a while and then the mole will disappear.

MULTIPLE SCLEROSIS

MS is the result of a lack of gold which causes a glandular imbalance. The lack of digestive ability or assimilation of gold is the chief physical disturbance in sclerosis conditions. This results in a hormonal deficiency/imbalance, and thus disturbs proper functioning of the nerves.

Therapy:
•Massage the body daily with combination of: 2 ounces olive and 2 ounces peanut oil with 1/4 ounce lanolin - supportive therapy muscles that have lost normal innervation.
•Vibrational therapy to reestablish proper physiological function (device provided in consultation)
•Enlightened Athletics Dietary Protocol with addition of B-complex vitamin (including adenosylcobalamin); Brewers yeast; water crest; carrots; celery; beets; salad and vegetables with gelatin; fruits; cereals; and avoid meats.

MUSCULAR DYSTROPHY

Primarily a glandular malfunction with a secondary effect on the motor nerves to the muscles, and a tertiary result in the muscular tissue. It often originates with a karmic etiology and occurs when the glandular activity breaks down at any point and the rest of the body is called upon in an abnormal manner and the substances required aren't supplied.

Begin with a spiritual attitude
Suggested Reading: Deuteronomy 30; John 14-17

Therapy:
•Enlightened Athletics Dietary Protocol with no red meat
•Nascent iodine, which purifies the glands and is both curative and preventative
•Assist the nerve tissue of the body in gaining strength and vitality with vibratory device (provided in consult)
•Massage for at least 30 minutes with constructive affirmations, using equal amounts of olive oil and peanut oil

NARCOLEPSY

A subtle disturbance, resulting in an inability to remain conscious of reactions or responses between the brain and sensory forces. It is associated with a blood disturbance, specifically a lack of effluvia.

Therapy:
•Enlightened Athletics Dietary Protocol with emphasis on foods rich in iron, vitamin A, vitamin D, and vitamin B1
•Hydrotherapy Colonics
•Witch hazel vapor baths
•Vibrational treatments to regenerate and coordinate nervous systems

NEUROPATHY

Formed by pressures upon nerves which lead to in-coordinate reactions.

Common Causes:
Diabetes mellitus - due to changes caused by high blood sugar levels
Shingles - can result in nerve damage
Vitamin deficiency
Alcohol
Toxin exposure
Inherited disorder

Therapy:
•Enlightened Athletics Dietary Protocol with emphasis on spinach, celery, peas, berries, fruits, carrots, lettuce, cabbage and lentils
•Regular Swedish massage using olive oil and tincture of myrrh; massage from central portion of the body and work toward extremities. Work to relax and contract the muscular forces and focus where cerebrospinal and sympathetic nerve forces coordinate, extending from below the thyroid to the pubic area on the front of the body, and from the base of the brain to the coccyx on the back side of the body.
•Daily massage following the nerves toward their end from the ninth dorsal upwards towards the hands, and from the ninth dorsal downwards towards the feet.
•Vibrational treatments to regenerate and coordinate nervous systems

OBESITY

Etiology is found in an excess of starches creating a hardening of the glandular system as well as tissues of the small intestinal wall, and thus changing the nature of those cells which absorb and metabolize carbohydrates. A radical change in diet is necessary to bring about changes in the cells of the intestinal tract which will reverse the tendency of those cells to turn most things into sugar.

Correct the diet and restore balance and efficiency with:
•Enlightened Athletics Dietary Protocol

Balance the glandular system, especially the adrenals and pineal gland with:
•nascent iodine

Ensure adequate eliminations:
•proper hydration
•senna laxative
•regular enemas

Correct other abnormalities; nervous system incoordination, circulatory system imbalance, etc., which can create conditions conducive to excess body weight:
•massage
•osteopathic manipulation

PARKINSON'S

Most commonly caused by an incoordination in the nervous system initiated at the glandular level in the patches of the emunctory circulation that controls coordination between sympathetic and cerebrospinal nerve systems. Additionally, it may be brought on by mercury poisoning, medication, or infection.

The object is to reestablish the coordination between the nervous systems and stimulate the glands with the process of regeneration, using both massage which directly and reflexively benefits both the circulatory and nervous system, and the use of a vibrational device provided in consult.

Therapy:
•Enlightened Athletics Dietary Protocol with extra calcium-rich foods
•Nascent iodine
•Massage the body with either olive oil or peanut oil
•Regular general osteopathic or chiropractic adjustments
•Regular use of vibrational device

PROSTATE CANCER

The aim is to balance and coordinate physiological functions and bring about a greater Oneness between body, mind, and spirit.

Common causes:
Resentments; Nervous system incoordination; Excess uric acid in bloodstream; Disturbance in the assimilations and/or eliminations

Therapy:
•Enlightened Athletics Dietary Protocol add sprouted almonds
•Osteopathic Adjustments especially to cervical; upper and mid dorsal; and sacrococcygeal outflow of nerves
•Massage especially to the sacrococcygeal region
•Hydrotherapy colonic
•Application of sodium bicarbonate solution applied to sacrum and both sides of the gland in groin massaged in well
•Application of a hot sea salt pack to the area

PROSTATITIS

Caused by infection or nerve reflex, but invariably other organs of the digestive and elimination systems are involved in the etiology, and thus a local and general regard to causation and treatment is required.

Regarding the non-infectious nerve reflex prostatitis, reflex involves the lower area of the spine and transmitted via the ileum plexus, the nerve ganglia associated with pelvic organs and reproductive system.

Therapies:

•Enlightened Athletics Dietary Protocol emphasizing fresh fruits and vegetables
•Hydrotherapy colonics
•Senna laxatives
•General and Prostate massage
•Sitz bath
•Castor oil pack over abdomen

PYORRHEA

The action of this particular bacilli is first finding a site for growth and multiplication, either by invasive action or by predisposing conditions. The organism has the same shape of a bedbug but with larger legs.

Therapy:
•Massage gums thoroughly and vigorously with a liberal quantity of ipsab, rinse with an undiluted solution of Glyco-Thymoline and then with water thereafter
•Brush teeth each evening with combination of equal parts salt and baking soda.
•Enlightened Athletics Dietary Protocol with a large raw salad each day

SCARS

Let the scars be removed from your mental and spiritual self.

Therapy for the removal of cutaneous scars:

Massage in alternation a camphorated olive oil (using natural gum found in Cinnamomum Camphor) around and on the affected area; and olive oil with tincture of myrrh (heat olive oil before adding tincture, and make just enough for each application). The olive oil will stimulate muscular and mucous membrane activity, while the myrrh acts with the pores to bring circulation to affected parts; and the camphorated oil brings a soothing stimulation in such a way to bring about new skin.

The whole surface of the skin can be changed if this protocol is followed persistently and consistently over 2.5 years.

SEXUAL FULFILLMENT

Examine and set your ideals and values, and so keep yourself unspotted from the world. Let sex never be for only emotional satisfaction, but creative in nature. There is no condemnation in having sex, unless it be for personal, selfish gratification.

Sexuality enhances growth if the deepest motive is to find Oneness of all Life. Sexuality is the arena where we can uncover the fundamental oneness of all energy. This doesn't always mean gratification in the physical act, but creativity in general, as sexual expression is a movement of creative force.

When sexual ecstasy takes us outside of ourselves, that spiritual experience is of the highest vibration in the material world, and is a state very similar to that state of consciousness accompanying a kundalini awakening. Great growth can be made spiritually with the right ideal cast and values set in sexuality.

Souls must assert their Light to know they are Light.

SHINGLES

The Thoracic area, Cervical, Lumbar, Sacral, and 5th Cranial Nerve are most commonly involved.

This malaise is not of an infectious etiology, but of a basic pathology, involving at its root poor eliminations initiated by a variety of mechanisms, brought about by a hydrochloric portion of the system, and by series of effect is there only an apparent virus attack with characteristic distribution around spinal or cranial nerves reflecting the segments innervated by the involved nerves.

Therapy:
•Enlightened Athletics Dietary Protocol; easily digestible; no apples, sweets, or meat; supplement Vitamin B-1; drink Watermelon Seed Tea to stimulate eliminations
•Osteopathic Adjustments with emphasis on dorsal, cervical, and lumbar
•Massage Peanut Oil mixed in equal parts with Witch Hazel

SINUSITIS

Not a local infection but a general condition which finds expression in the soft tissue or mucous membranes where lymph is circulated.

Pressures on spinal nerves are the primary factor and commonly found in the upper dorsals and cervicals. Irritants occur through a combination of poor circulation, poor elimination, and acid-alkaline imbalance. The irritants make for an allergic effect. Associated indigestion caused by absorption of mucus in G.I. tract.

Therapy:
•Osteopathic adjustments
•Enlightened Athletics Dietary Protocol
•Hydrotherapy (colonic irrigation)
•General Massage
•Nascent iodine

Acute symptom relief: Saturate in glycothymoline a cotton cloth of 2 to 3 sheets thickness, and wrap around facial sinuses - apply for two hours.

Less acute symptom relief: Mix glycothymoline and distilled water for use as a nasal spray

STREPTOCOCCUS

The usual cause of the streptococcus attacking vulnerable parts of the body is nervous strain. Fundamental to recovery is an attitude shift.

Therapy:
•Enlightened Athletics Dietary Protocol
•Hydrotherapy Colonic or Enema
•Formula: 20 minims of camphor gum; 20 minims of muriated iron; 1/2 grain of sulphate of morphia. Mix together. Divide into 20 pellets. Take 1 up to twice a day with 2 hours between each dose.
•Inhalant: 4 oz pure grain alcohol; 30 minims eucalyptol; 5 minims rectified oil of turpentine; 5 minims Canadian balsam; 30 minims tolu solution. Shake before use. Inhale every hour or every few minutes until irritation is allayed.

STUTTERING

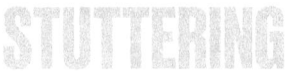

Reduction of the tendency of the body to oversupply energy to the vocal cords is required. The connections for the auditory as well as the vocal forces of the body derive their impulse from the 3rd cervical, as well as the 3rd, 4th, and 5th dorsal. Correct the subluxations and and pressures along the spine, and ensure a good and patient attitude.

Therapy:
•2-3 osteopathic adjustments per week until resolved (adequate adjustments are necessary, lest the problem recur)
•Spinal massage with peanut oil

SUNBURNS

One of the greatest enemies to a beautiful complexion is too much sunshine. During the period of 11-14.00 there is too great a quantity of actinic rays for the superficial circulation of the skin. Early mornings and late afternoons are the preferred times to enjoy the sun and prevent overexposure.

Aloe vera may be great to use in a pinch, but for a more complete treatment there is nothing better than pure apple vinegar. Apply it to the affected area as a balm or lotion.

Therapy for acute breakouts resulting from sunburn: Daub the affected area with spirits of camphor using cotton balls; two hours after application enjoy a tepid bath; then apply peanut oil.

TONSILLITIS

Tonsils are for the normal healthy development and necessary to the body - relieving tension and strain in the system. Tonsillitis, the impairment of circulation, either generally or locally as the throat seeks to bring about equilibrium, results from wastes and toxins in the circulation. Underlying every condition of inflamed tonsils or adenoids are inadequate eliminations, either generally or locally. Associated and often causative are lesions and subluxations in the cervical or upper dorsal which impede function in the circulation of the throat and head.

Approach as therapeutic problem with the whole person in view. The aim is to bring about adequate eliminations through all channels; purify and clarity the blood and intestinal tract. Correct pressures and lesions which may be present in upper vertebrae

Therapy:
•Do not strain the throat or body
•Enlightened Athletics Dietary Protocol
•Osteopathic adjustments
•Hydrotherapy Colonics and Enemas

Ulcers are brought about primarily by disturbances in digestion, assimilation, and elimination. Specific causes reduce to this basic triad - one system affecting the other. Treat the distressing symptoms knowing that often individual treatment of symptoms will be unnecessary if the underlying problems are addressed, since they are of a reflex origin.

Therapy:
- Hydrotherapy Colonics (every other day)
- Osteopathic adjustment especially the 3rd-5th dorsals
- Massages twice a week, using heated olive oil with tincture of myrrh
- Enlightened Athletics Dietary Protocol with added citrus juices and digestive aids; no apples, tuberous vegetables, bananas, or acid-producing fruits.
- Yellow saffron tea
- Castor oil packs (daily)
- Avoid excessive strain on the nervous system through proper mental and emotional outlook — avoid stress and rest

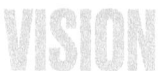

VISION

Stimulate optic reactions between kidneys and eyes with a whole carrot blended and mixed into gelatin and consumed with other above ground vegetables in at least one daily salad.

Therapy:
•Enlightened Athletics Dietary Protocol added carrots, green peas, green beans, onions, beets, oranges, lemons, limes. Prepare the vegetables and fruits with gelatin (especially the carrot) to increase absorption and directly aid the optic nerve
•Neck exercises - 3 relaxed head tilts to all sides, 3 clockwise head rolls, followed by 3 counterclockwise rolls
•Walk for at least 30 minutes each morning
•Remove the pressure of toxic forces by using an organic potato skin to create a poultice and cover your eyes with it for 20 minutes

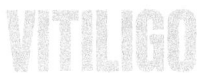

VITILIGO

A glandular disturbance effecting superficial circulation of skin reflected upon the liver where, along with the kidneys, inadequate function leads to toxins that should be eliminated through the alimentary canal or urine, but which end up in the skin.

Therapy:
•Enlightened Athletics Dietary Protocol
•Nascent iodine
•Ragweed tonic
•Hydrotherapy Colonic
•Castor oil enema

VAGUS NERVE

Coordinate the 2nd and 3rd dorsal for a general stimulation and regulating impulse to the vagus nerve. Anatomical correction should first be considered, followed by regulation of physiological function. They needn't be disassociated though as they may both occur in the same treatment.

Conditions of irritability and nervousness may be replaced with a normal and natural condition. Regulate vasomotor area then regulate the 4th and 8th dorsal. The first will regulate circulation and the second will equalize secretion.

By first adjusting the atlas, the pneumo-gastric nervous system and phrenic system are effected. By adjustment of the upper cervical, the vasomotor area, circulation of blood and all other bodily fluids are regulated. From the 1st to 4th dorsal influence is had over the pyloric end of the stomach and the lungs; 4th to 12th influence is had over the abdominal viscera; with further regulation by the dorsal and lumbar nerves.

LIGHT TOOLS

Gems and stones are just stepping stones, not foundations. Light Tools are lights upon the way to help in helping others. They provide orderly vibrations to quicken the spirit and help brighten the way for another.

Thy Light is the Great Light

AMETHYST

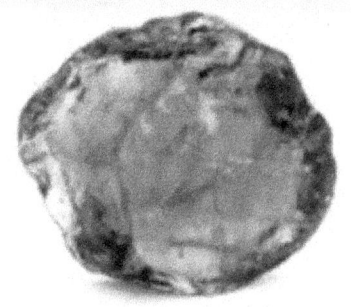

VIBRATIONS THAT BALANCE ENERGETIC CENTERS AND INFLUENCE SPIRITUAL DEVELOPMENT AND EXPRESSIONS IN ASSOCIATIONS

LIGHT TOOLS

LAPIS LAZULI

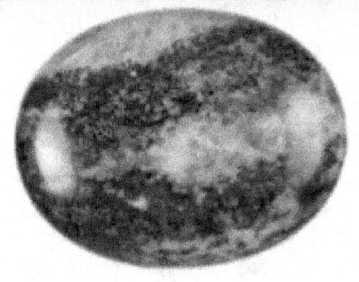

STRENGTHENS THE BODY AND ADAPTIVELY ENHANCES PSYCHIC ABILITY IN THE MANNER ONE IS SEEKING

LIGHT TOOLS

GOLD

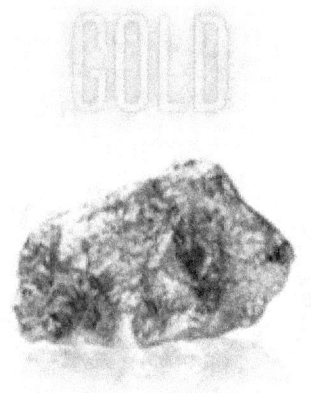

VIBRATIONS OF STRENGTH

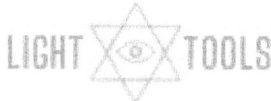

LARIMAR

POTENT HEALING VIBRATIONS

LIGHT TOOLS

SILVER

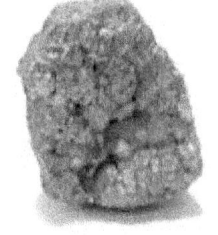

VIBRATIONS OF STABILITY

LIGHT TOOLS

COPPER

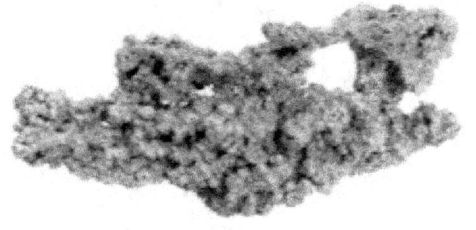

VIBRATIONS OF PASSION AND INTENSITY

LIGHT ✡ TOOLS

CORAL

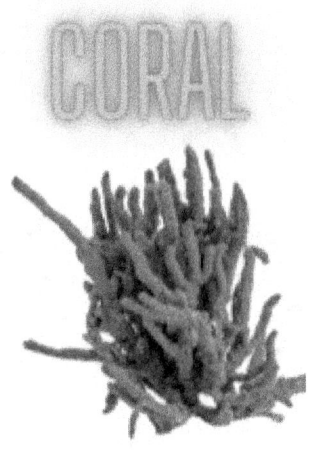

SYMPATHETIC WITH NATURE'S VIBRATIONS

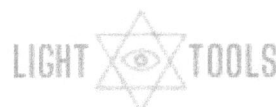

DIAMOND

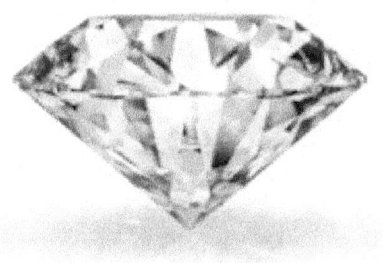

ATTUNES TO THE INFINITE. IT CAN FIRE
SELFISH IMAGINATION OR BRING PEACE

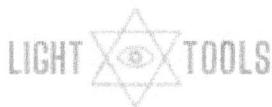

LIGHT TOOLS

PEARL

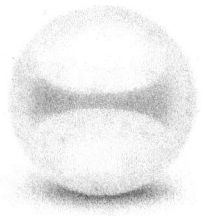

A BEAUTY WROUGHT BY HARDSHIPS,
OVERCOME THAT LENDS ITSELF TO HEALING,
CREATIVITY, PHYSICAL EXERCISE, AND
STRENGTHENING OF POISE

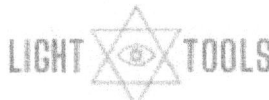

LIGHT TOOLS

BLOODSTONE

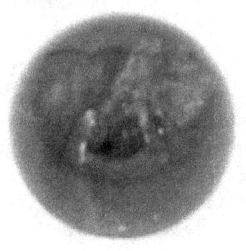

VIBRATIONS OF A HELPFUL FORCE PHYSICALLY THAT ENCOURAGE AND INFLUENCE THE MIND TOWARDS HARMONY

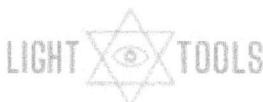

LIGHT TOOLS

AZURITE

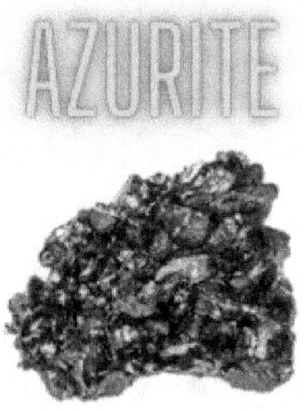

A TOUCHSTONE FOR THOSE INTERESTED IN THE
PSYCHIC THAT INDUCES INFLUENCES FROM
WITHOUT TO AID AN INDIVIDUAL IN CONTACT
WITH HIGHER SOURCES OF ACTIVITY

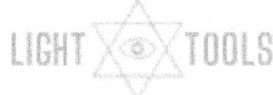

LIGHT TOOLS

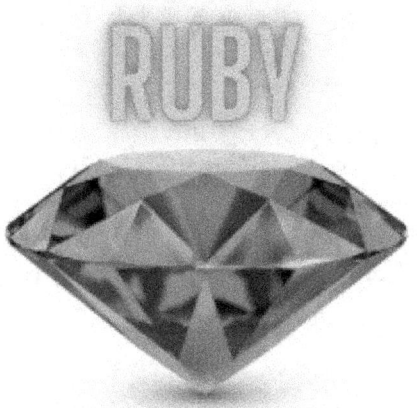

RUBY

VIBRATIONS THAT ENABLE A GREATER ABILITY TO CONCENTRATE MENTAL ENERGIES INTO MATERIAL EXPRESSION

LIGHT TOOLS

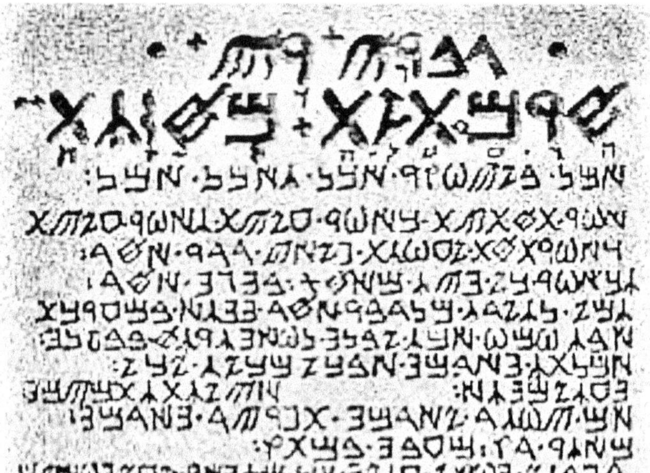

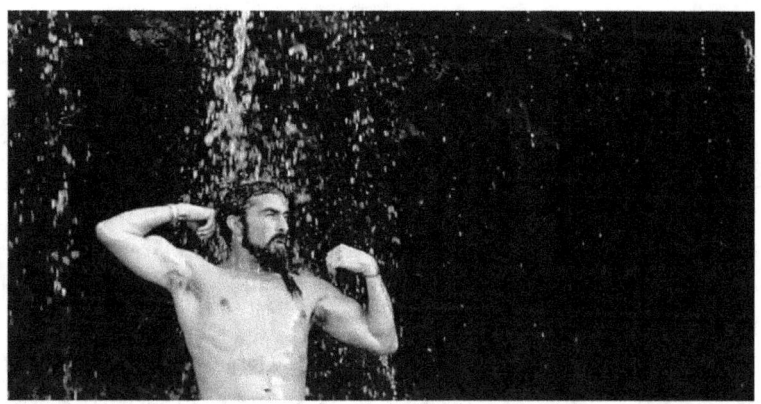

DONALD HOWBERT, DPM

'GLORIFY GOD, HONOR SELF'

ITINERANT MINISTER, HEALER,
COACH, AND RETREAT HOST

SON OF LIGHT MINISTRY

ENLIGHTENED ATHLETICS HIGH
PERFORMANCE INSTITUTE

GOODHELM TOURS

REVELATION YOGA

PATTERNING THE PHYSIOLOGY
FOR IDEAL HEALTH

SOCIAL MEDIA

AMAZON
REVELATION YOGA

INSTAGRAM
@ENLIGHTENED.ATHLETICS

FACEBOOK
@ENLIGHTENEDATHLETICS1

LINKEDIN
IN/DONALD-HOWBERT

CONTACT

IAM@LUX.GURU
WWW.LUX.GURU
303-898-0744

ABOUT THE MINISTRY

A Global Ministry for the Revelation of Truth, LUX.guru - Son of Light Ministry and its subsidiaries Enlightened Athletics High Performance Institute, Revelation Yoga, and Goodhelm Tours exist to repattern the physiology for ideal health and higher states of consciousness and by so doing lift every soul into Heaven. As an itinerant ministry offering, Revelation Yoga is brought to all Truth seekers, while Enlightened Athletics High Performance Institute promotes a healthy and fit lifestyle, and Goodhelm Tours makes available health recovery cruises.

For a full list of offerings and to book the ministry for a speaking arrangement, be sure to connect with us on social media and message us at IAM@LUX.guru

ENLIGHTENED ATHLETICS

REVELATION YOGA

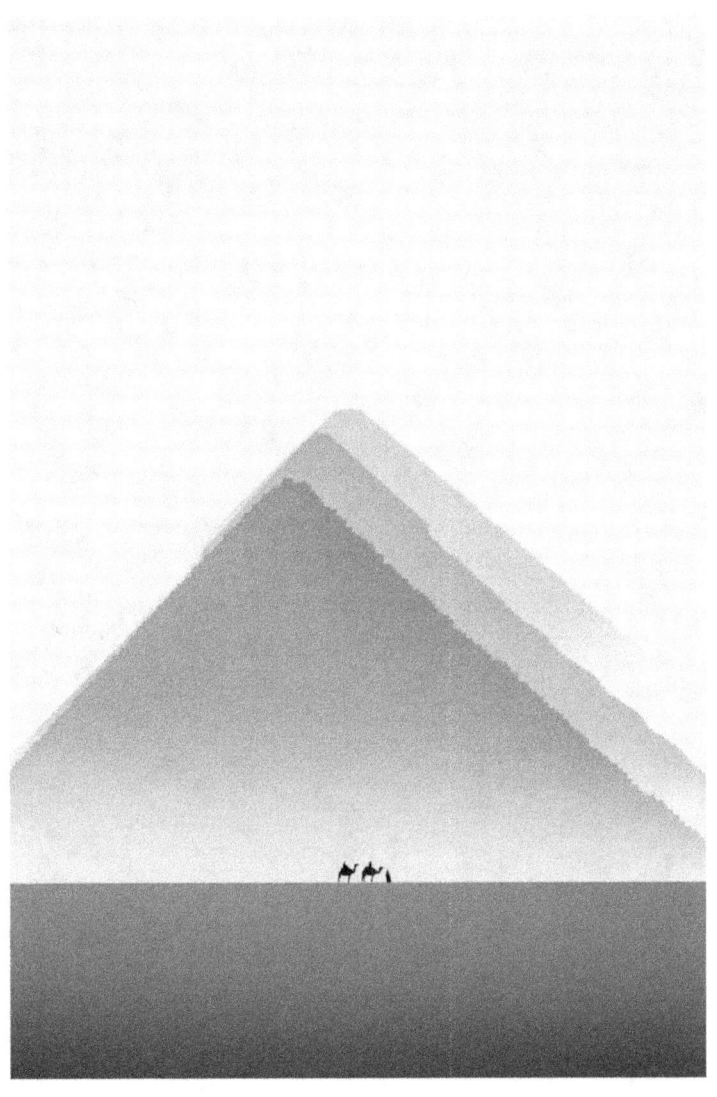

GOODHELM TOURS